8.29

Silent Dancer

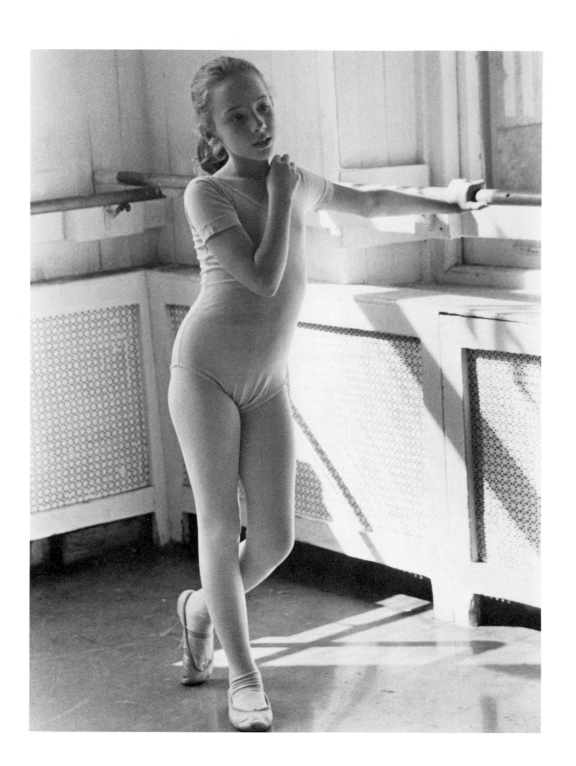

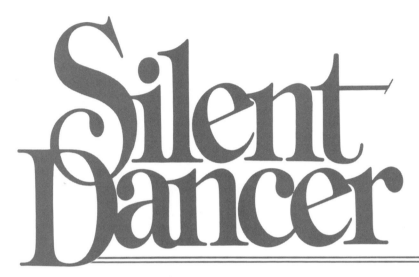

Silent Dancer

By Bruce Hlibok
Photographs by Liz Glasgow

JULIAN MESSNER   NEW YORK

Photographs on pages 22 & 23 courtesy of
Rehabilitation International, U.S.A.

Published by Julian Messner, a Simon & Schuster
Division of Gulf & Western Corporation,
Simon & Schuster Building,
1230 Avenue of the Americas,
New York, New York 10020.

JULIAN MESSNER and colophon are trademarks of
Simon & Schuster, registered in the U.S. Patent
and Trademark Office.

Library of Congress Cataloging in Publication Data

Hlibok, Bruce.
    Silent dancer.

    Summary: Text and photographs describe the
experiences of a ten-year-old deaf girl studying
ballet at the Joffrey Ballet School.
    1. Ballet—Juvenile literature.   2. Children,
Deaf—Recreation—Juvenile literature.   3. Joffrey
Ballet—Juvenile literature.   [1. Ballet dancing.
2. Deaf.   3. Physically handicapped.   4. Joffrey
Ballet]   I. Glasgow, Liz, ill.   II. Title.
GV1787.5.H54   792.8'2   81-14011

ISBN 0-671-43260-5   AACR2

Manufactured in the United States of America.

Design by Meri Shardin

For all children
with dreams

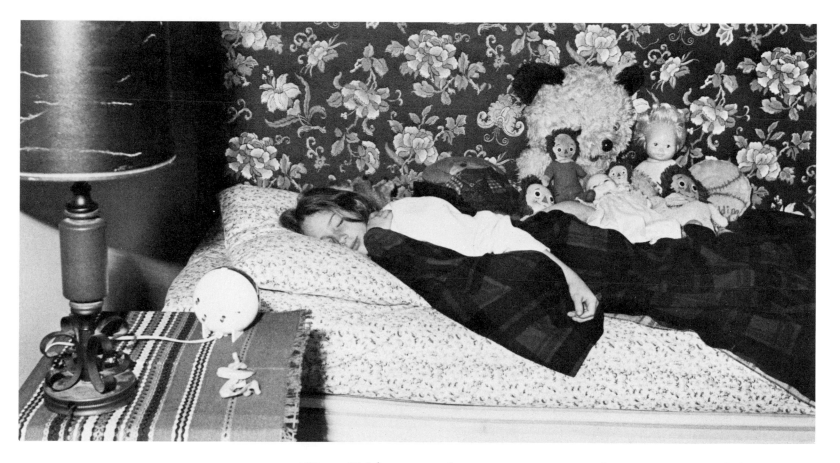

On Friday morning, as on every other morning of the week, ten-year-old Nancy wakes up when her alarm clock flashes on and off. Yes, *flashes*. Nancy has an alarm clock with a light that flashes on and off, instead of one that rings.

Nancy is deaf. She cannot hear most of the sounds in the world, but she uses her eyes in the way hearing people use their ears.

On the other mornings of the week when Nancy's alarm clock flashes, she groans and tries to go back to sleep. But on Friday Nancy comes wide awake. Friday is special, the best day of the week. Friday is the day she goes to ballet class.

7

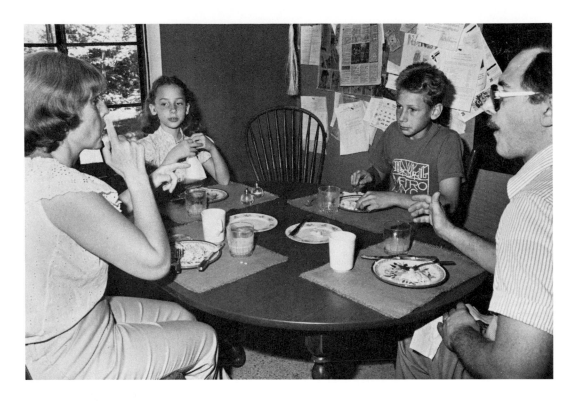

When she has washed and dressed, Nancy goes downstairs to the kitchen where her mother is making breakfast. In time, the whole family sits down around the kitchen table, eating eggs and bacon and drinking orange juice, milk, and coffee. All of them are animated, their faces lit up, their hands picking up a fork, knife, or cup.

Nancy's parents and brother are also deaf. They use sign language to communicate with one another. So the conversation around the kitchen table is lively but quiet. Liveliest of all is Nancy, as she tells her parents and her younger brother that it's the day she goes to ballet class.

But first, Nancy must spend the day at her regular school. And this thought makes her eat her breakfast faster.

As always, the school bus arrives before Nancy and her brother Greg have finished breakfast, and their mother rushes them out, carrying their books and lunch bags. Nancy dashes back into the house to pick up her ballet leotards, which she left behind in her hurry. She catches the bus just in time!

Nancy has many friends on the bus. They are on their way to the Lexington School for the Deaf in New York City. All of them seem more lively because they are laughing and shouting and are talking with their hands at the same time. The children can even laugh with their hands.

Nancy is in the fourth grade. Her class with Ms. Byrnes is very small. The first thing Nancy has to do before class starts is to check that her hearing aids are working so that she can hear the teacher's voice. Nancy wears two self-contained hearing aids.

Each hearing aid is a small device that fits onto Nancy's ear. Each aid is really a tiny microphone that is hooked up to a miniature loudspeaker. The loudspeaker makes sounds louder so that Nancy can recognize them.

When Nancy was small, some of her neighborhood friends made fun of the "two lumps" behind her ears. It often upset her. But her parents always told her that it was important that she practice listening. Now Nancy finds her friends respect her and don't laugh at her anymore.

Nancy starts her day at school with speech class. Her speech teacher, Ms. Hunold, knows very well that Friday is the day Nancy goes to ballet class. Nancy talks of nothing but ballet every day.

"Ballet is pronounced 'ba-lay.' You should never say the *t* at the end of the word. 'Ballet' is a French word, and many French words end in a *t* that is silent."

Nancy watches and listens carefully as Ms. Hunold says the word.

"Ba-lay."

The teacher leans closer to Nancy's hearing aid and repeats the word. Nancy listens and watches the teacher's mouth to see the correct formations of the lips and tongue. Nancy repeats the word again and again to memorize the lip and tongue movements and the way it sounds. A biofeedback machine lights up when a letter sounds perfect. Sometimes Ms. Hunold covers Nancy's eyes, and Nancy repeats the word to see if she can say it without relying on the biofeedback panel.

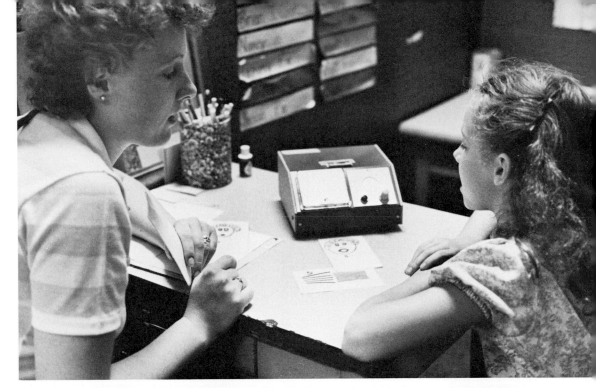

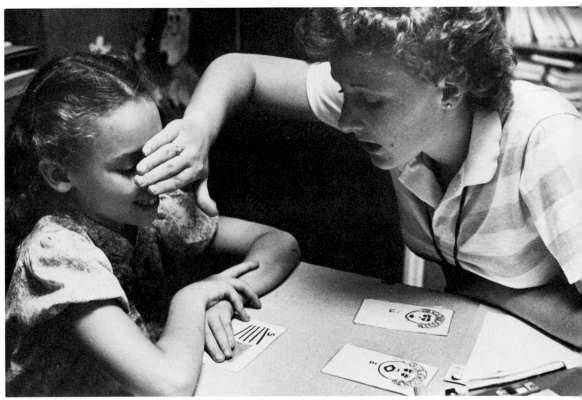

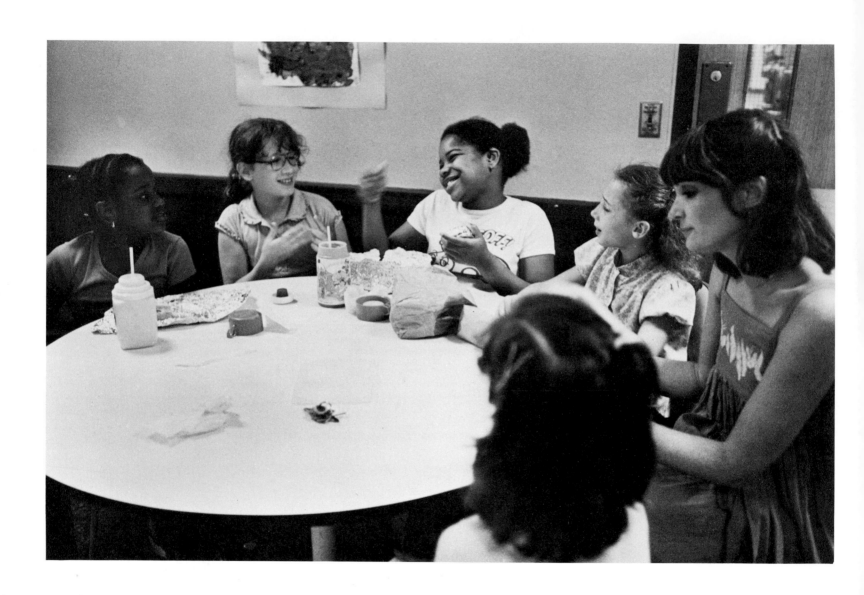

After math class, it is time for lunch. At lunch, Nancy sits with some of her friends from ballet school. Ms. Byrnes joins them. At lunchtime they can all have fun together. Ms. Byrnes asks Nancy if she finds it hard to wait for the end of the school day. Everyone laughs.

"Ballet class seems such a long time off," Nancy says. "I wish it was three already so that we could go! I'm tired of waiting."

Nancy peeks into her lunch bag, wrinkles her nose, and groans. Mother has packed tuna-fish sandwiches and raisins and an apple. Nancy would rather have peanut-butter and jelly sandwiches and some chocolate cake.

But Nancy knows that mother has done the right thing, for apples and raisins are more healthful to eat than cake. A dancer needs to eat well to have a strong body. Chocolate cake is delicious, but it does not make one strong enough for long hours of hard ballet practice.

After lunch, Nancy and her friend Krista go to the gym, where they do stretching exercises. Then Nancy has science class. She works with a classmate, looking at slides of different animal cells and writing down their names and descriptions. They try to pronounce some of the names, such as *amoeba,* a single-cell animal, and Ms. Byrnes helps by correcting their pronunciation.

A spelling bee comes next. Nancy has fun spelling words. There is lots of laughter in the class when someone misspells a word. Before Nancy realizes, it is already three o'clock. Ms. Byrnes tells the class that school is over.

Cleaning up her desk, Nancy packs her knapsack with schoolbooks she will need to do her assignments. She rushes out to the hall, where she meets Krista and the other girls who are going to ballet class. They all board a bus that takes them to Greenwich Village, where the Joffrey Ballet School is located.

The Joffrey Ballet School teaches children and young people ballet dancing. Many students have graduated from the school and gone on to join famous ballet companies all over the world.

When Nancy arrives at the ballet school, she goes straight to the dressing room. In the dressing room many girls are changing from their school clothes into leotards. Nancy changes into white tights and a sky blue leotard.

The girls, like all dancers, wear leotards in ballet class. The leotards stretch and make it easier for the students to move freely, and they show the lines of their legs and body.

Nancy also has to tie her hair back so that her neck will show and her hair will not fall into her eyes. When Nancy ties back her hair, her hearing aids show, but she does not care. Wearing her hearing aids is more important than her appearance.

After she is dressed, she picks up her ballet slippers. Her slippers are made of shiny pink satin, with an elastic band over the top. When she bought the slippers, Nancy sewed the elastic on herself because the slipper must fit each foot snugly so that it won't fall off.

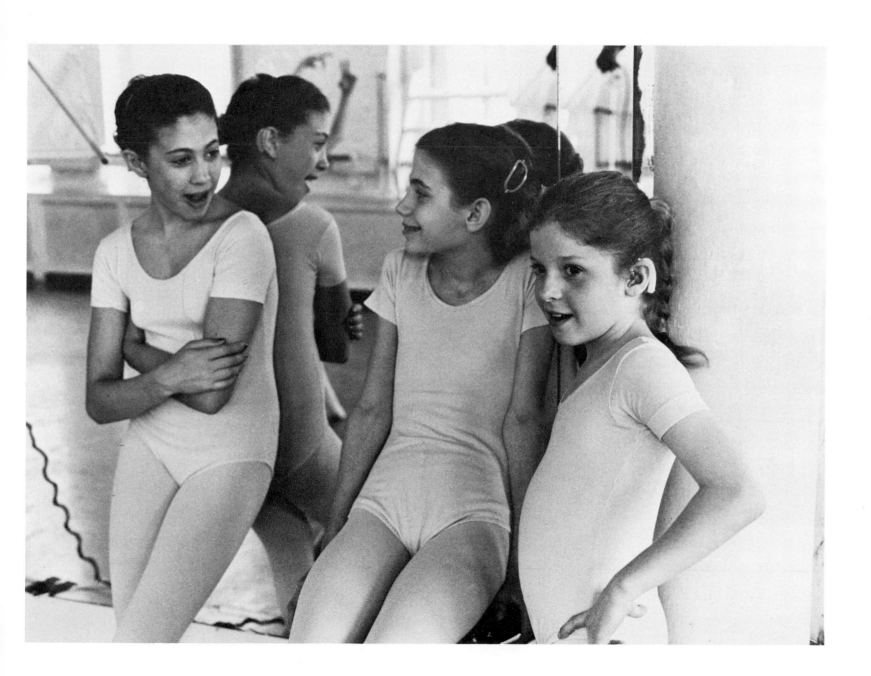

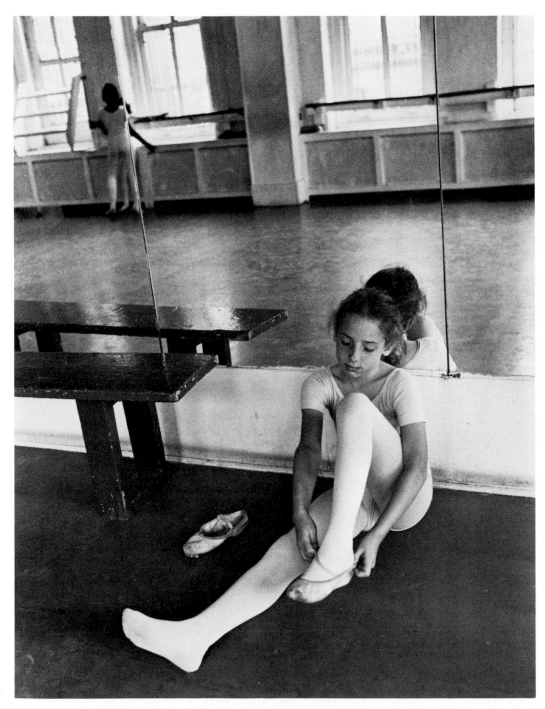

In the rehearsal studio, Nancy greets the other girls, and sitting down on the floor she puts on her slippers. The soles of her slippers are a little rough, in order to prevent her from slipping on the smooth floor. As she puts on her slippers, Nancy thinks back to the night about a year before when she was in the dressing room at Lincoln Center, putting on her costume to dance.

She was going to dance in a special event, a benefit to raise money to help handicapped children all over the world. Nancy and the other girls in the class for deaf children at the Joffrey School had learned a special dance for the show.

The program took place in the evening. Lincoln Center was crowded. People were jumping out of taxis and rushing into the great white marble buildings to concerts, operas, and ballets. In the center of the plaza a fountain lit by colored lights shot up water into changing patterns. Through the glass fronts of the theaters colorful paintings and gold sculptures shone brightly into the night. The lobbies were filled with lively groups of people dressed in party clothes.

Backstage, everything was in chaos. People were running back and forth, changing lights and sets, and dancers were exercising near a wall. The stage manager was telling everybody what to do.

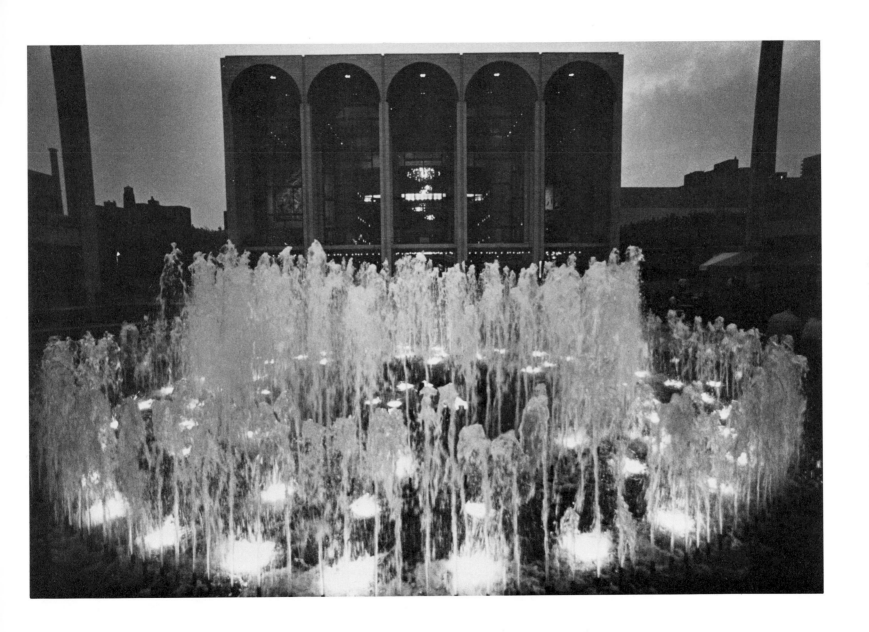

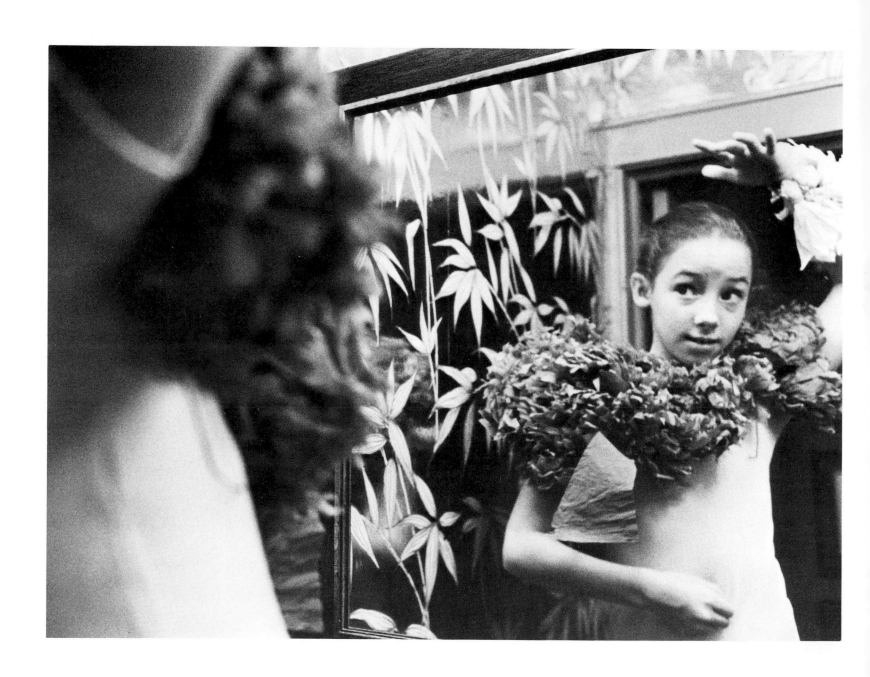

In the dressing room there was an air of excitement. People helped Nancy to get ready, to comb her hair and get into a costume made especially for her.

The girls were nervous because they had never seen so many people in a theater or so many things happening at once. But they forgot their nervousness when they saw themselves in the mirrors. Their costumes were made of many layers of pink and red satin. They looked like the little flower elves they were supposed to be. Before Nancy knew it, she and the others were rushed to a place where they could go on stage as soon as the curtain went up.

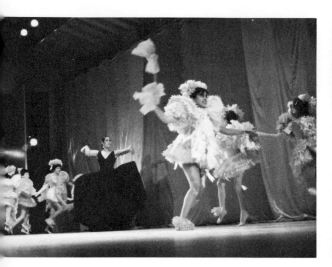

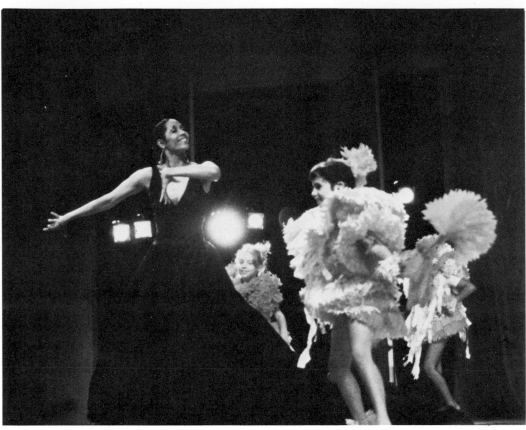

A famous actress announced that the next dance was a special one because the young dancers were deaf. The audience clapped, and then as the lights went down, everything became quiet.

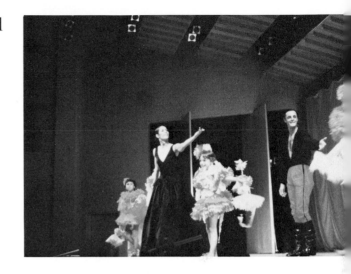

The music started, the curtain rose, and the lights went up. One thousand people applauded as Nancy and her classmates danced on stage. The applause was so loud that Nancy could feel it. Two grown-up ballet dancers came on, and the dance began.

The dance was about a flower princess and a prince who loved her. But the flower princess had many flower elves— Nancy and her classmates—who kept playing tricks on the prince, keeping him away from the princess. The flower elves were perfect, and Nancy felt fine. She was doing everything right, and she had a feeling of pride in her body. She moved to the music, her feet skipping and turning. She knew now that she wanted to be a dancer!

Finally the prince outdid the elves, kissed the princess, and that made a happy ending. After the dance was over, the curtain came down and went right back up, because the audience was applauding loudly. The prince and princess gestured to the flower elves who had to curtsy many, many times before they finally got off the stage.

Backstage, everybody was hugging and kissing the children, and Nancy had never felt so proud of herself.

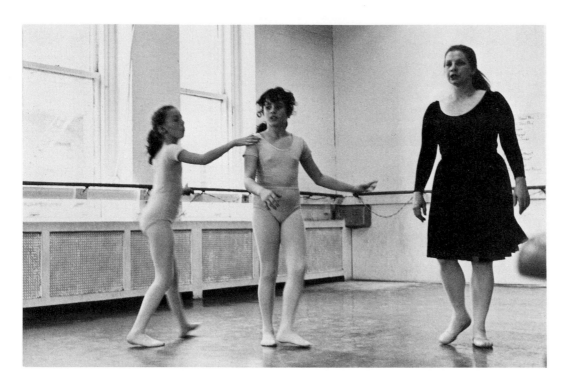

Nancy gets up quickly as her teacher, Ms. Meredith Baylis, comes into the studio to start this week's class at the Joffrey School. She walks slowly around the room to make sure that every girl is prepared. She wants all the girls to look their best and wants to know that they feel comfortable in their leotards. If a student feels uncomfortable, she will find it hard to concentrate on her exercises.

Ms. Baylis works with the other ballet teachers on the faculty of the Joffrey Ballet School. She was a leading ballerina with a famous American-based ballet company, the Ballet Russe de Monte Carlo, for many years. The company traveled all over the United States, Canada, and South America. The girls know her well because she has been teaching the class for three years, and most of the girls have been with her all that time.

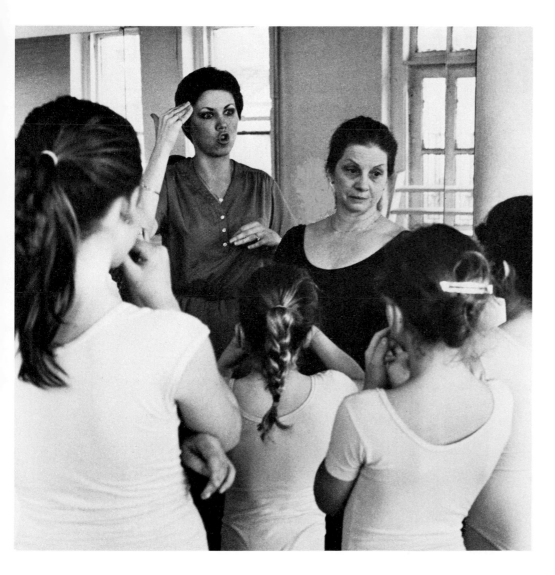

Helping her in the class is Marianne Gluszak, an interpreter/
aide. Marianne's job is to sign in sign language what Ms.
Baylis says to the students and to talk for some of the students
whose speech is not always easily understood.

25

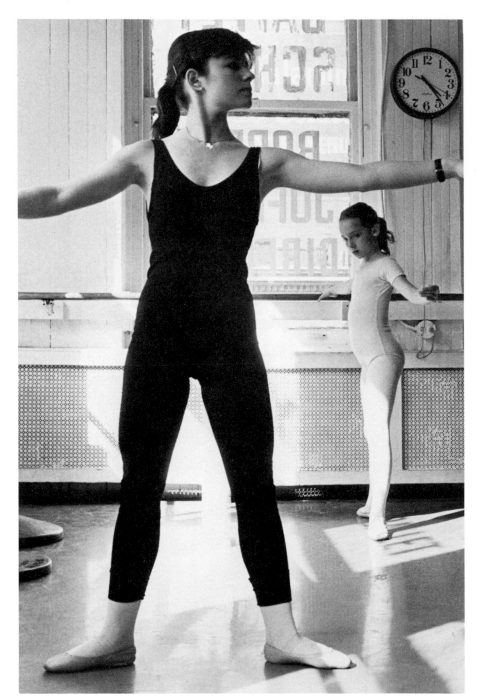
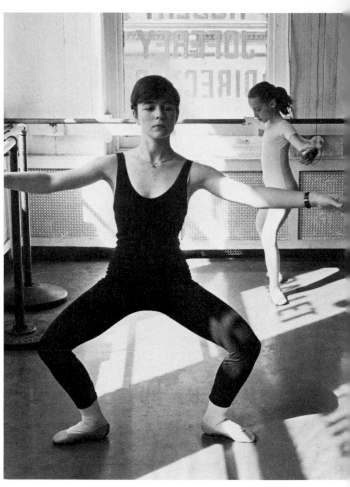

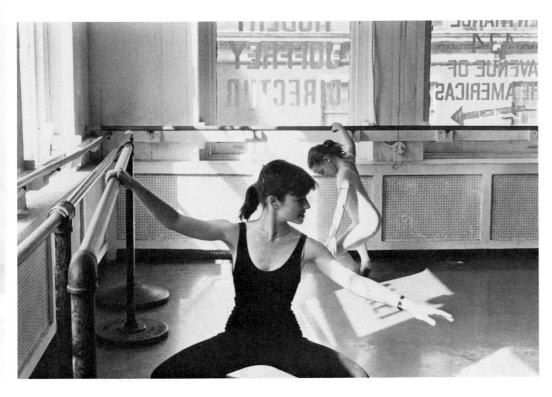

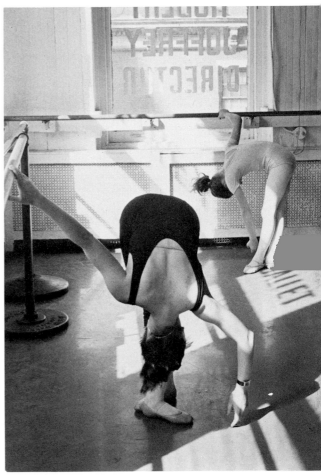

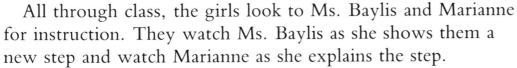

All through class, the girls look to Ms. Baylis and Marianne for instruction. They watch Ms. Baylis as she shows them a new step and watch Marianne as she explains the step.

A hearing teenager, Lauren Evans, an advanced ballet student who knows some sign language, acts as a demonstrator. She shows the class how to do a step correctly while the teacher points out the proper body movements.

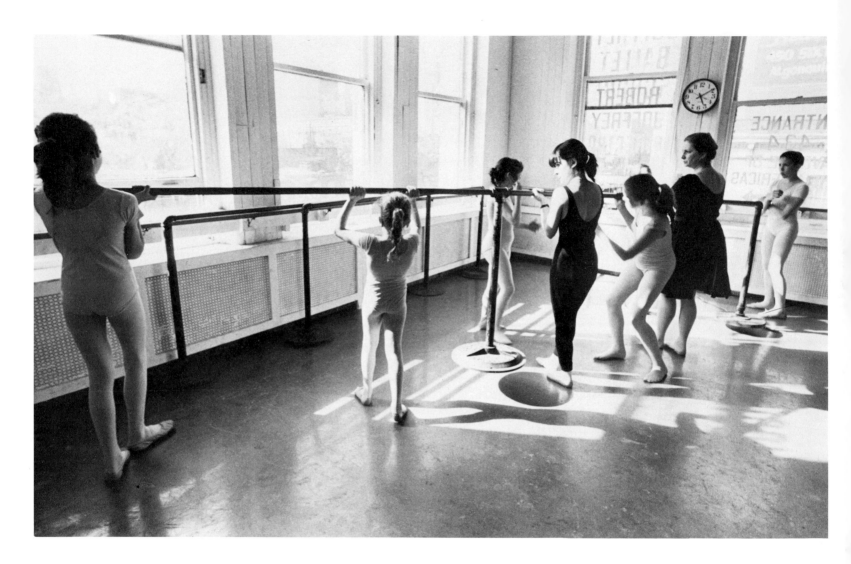

The rehearsal studio is a long white room with mirrors along one wall and windows in two walls overlooking the street. A long wooden pole runs along three sides of the room about four feet above the floor. This pole is called a *barre*. There are also movable *barres* that the class can put where they will have more space to move around. Every dancer uses a *barre* to learn how to balance properly.

There is a large piano in the studio. It is no ordinary piano, for it is connected to a special sound system. Two loudspeakers rest on the floor and make it vibrate with the sound. When the pianist plays some music, the sound is made louder by the speakers and the vibrations come through the floor so that the class can feel the music.

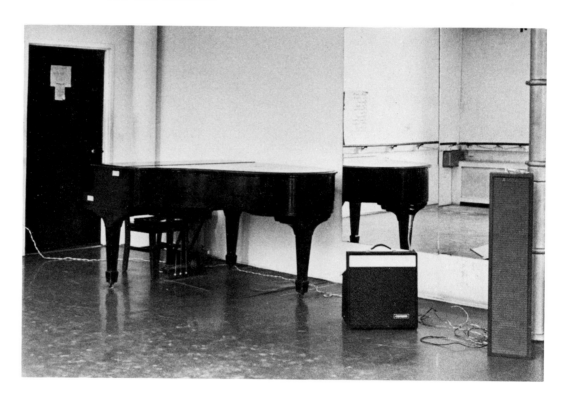

When Ms. Baylis first taught the class how to dance to music, she had the girls count out loud in groups of numbers, the way the music is played:

"One . . . two . . . three . . ." and the class would breathe and continue, "one . . . two . . . three . . ." and breathe again.

"Count eight! And breathe!" Ms. Baylis would say.

Class starts with the breathing exercises. Then they do a few stretching exercises before the real lesson begins.

Every girl who wants to be a ballerina always dreams of being able to dance "on toe." This means dancing with your feet and body balanced on your toes. Nancy and her classmates will eventually learn how to dance this way, but first they must learn how to balance properly and know most of the ballet movements.

Ballet dancing involves muscles of the body that are not used to the work asked of them. Muscles have to be trained and strengthened. "On toe" dancing requires very strong muscles in the legs. If it is taught too soon before the other exercises, it could damage leg muscles.

Dancing seems so easy, so effortless when you are watching ballerinas on stage, but what you are watching is the result of many years of long, hard work. It comes from strict training and a healthy body.

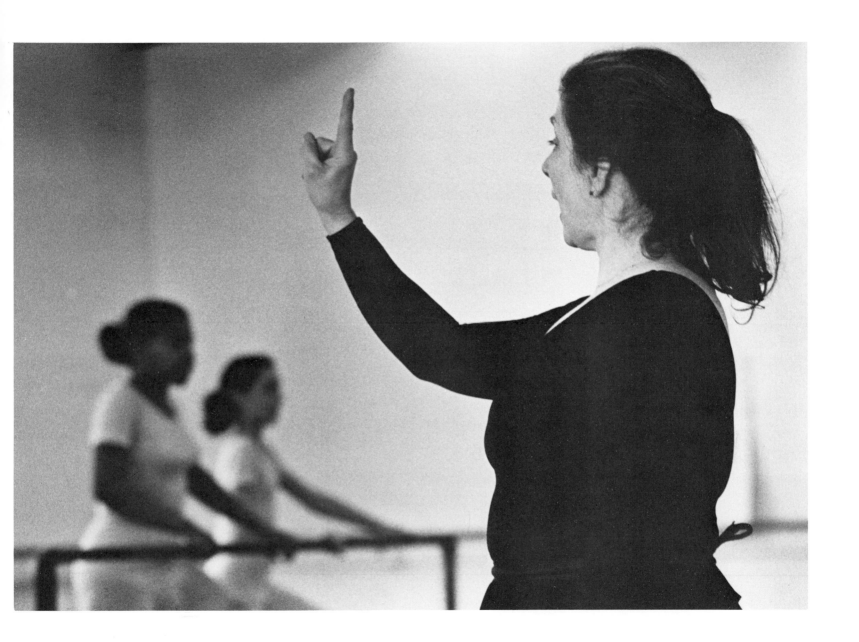

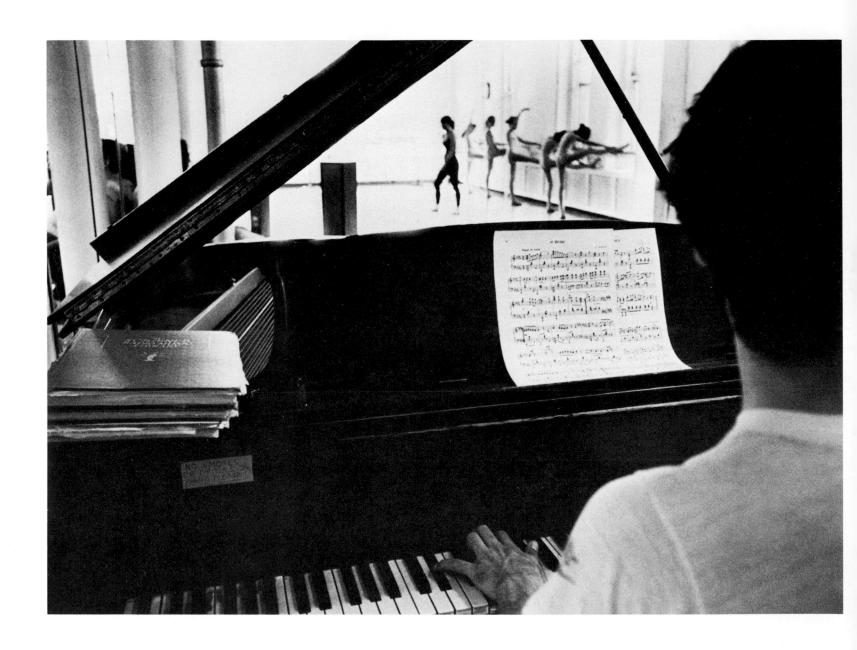

When the class is finished with the stretching exercises, Stefan Molinas, the pianist, starts playing some ballet music.

When Nancy rehearses, she always wears her hearing aids so she can get the most out of both hearing and feeling the music. This makes it easier for her to follow the dance steps.

Music helps put a sense of rhythm in the bodies of the girls. Ms. Baylis has each girl place her hand on the piano and feel the beat of the music as the pianist plays. She uses great care in picking out the musical compositions for the class. The rhythm of the music must be clear and easy to feel and understand. The music is often by Chopin, Drigo, and Minkus, who are famous for their dance music.

The class lines up at the *barre,* so that each one can see Ms. Baylis, Marianne, the demonstrator, and the mirrors all at the same time.

On one wall is a sign listing the ten basic ballet steps. This sign is used in all ballet classes to help the students remember the name of each ballet movement.

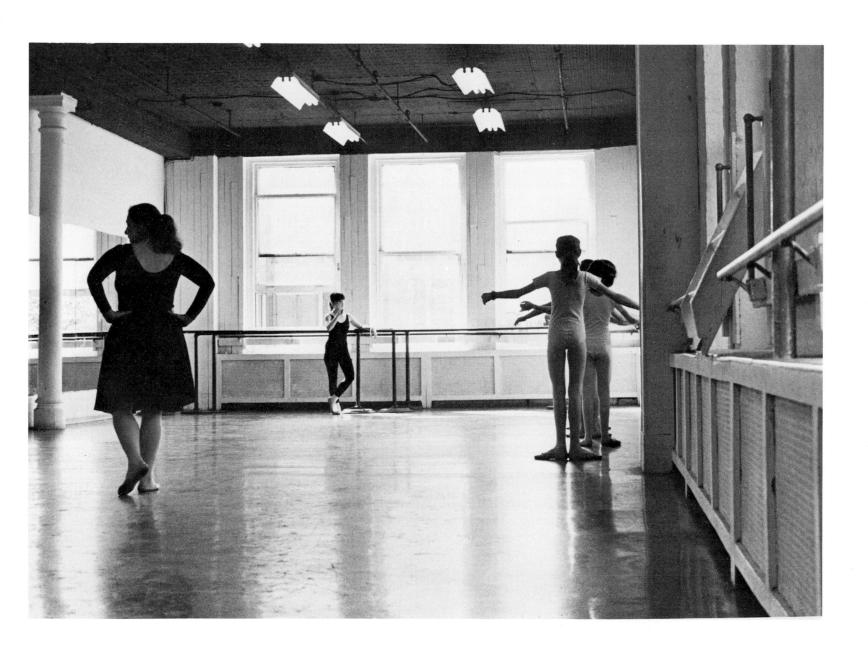

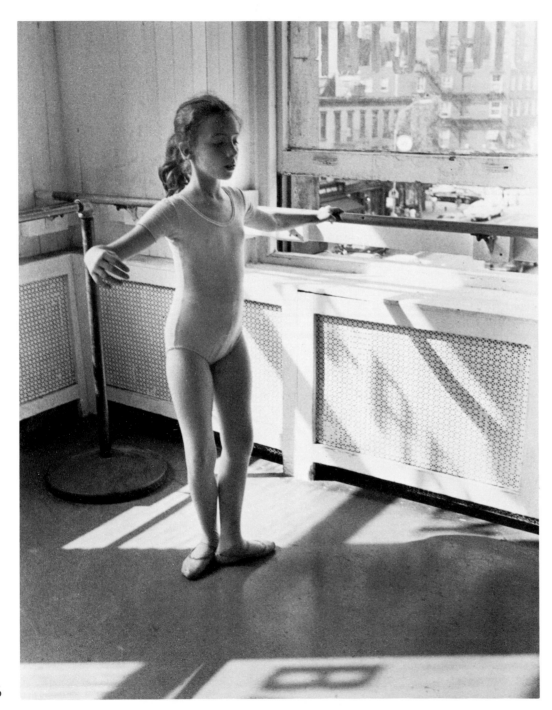

At first, the names seemed strange to Nancy, for the words are French. French is the language of the ballet. The French people were among the first to recognize ballet as a beautiful art form, and the first national ballet school was founded in France. By now Nancy knows which step each word means.

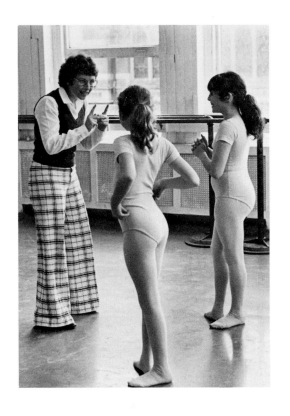

At the barre *I learn how to keep my legs in the right place. When I do this, I find it easier to follow the movements. There are five basic positions. I'm doing the third now.*

I stand beside the barre, *with my left hand on the* barre, *and I raise my right arm up, in a curve. My right hand is on the same level as my shoulders. I turn out my toes as far as I can while I keep my feet together. I use my whole leg to turn out my foot. Ms. Baylis said never to use the hips. I am supposed to keep my body straight, but sometimes my stomach sticks out a little.*

Nancy goes on to repeat the other four basic positions over and over. The second one involves the first position, and the third the second, and so forth. They are used in different combinations to form other ballet positions.

Ms. Judith Evans comes into the studio. She is a teacher of deaf children who first thought of having this ballet class. The Joffrey School agreed to try it, and the class has become a success. Ms. Evans likes to stop by to see the girls dancing and to encourage them to work hard.

The class continues doing the basic ballet movements. Each movement must be learned well because later they are put together to form complicated dances. The class has already learned most of the basic movements.

Just because they know some of the movements does not mean that they can stop practicing them, because more practice helps the dancer become more precise in each movement. It makes it possible to dance complicated dances, for one bad movement can spoil a whole dance. As the class goes along, they learn new movements while practicing the ones they learned before.

Now the class must practice fast turns down the long studio. They line up. It is time for Nancy to try. When she spins down the room, Ms. Baylis sees that she has held her arms in the wrong position.

The teacher stops Nancy and leads her to the mirrors. Holding Nancy's arms at the correct height, she tells her to notice that her hands are on the same level as her shoulders. Nancy looks at herself and understands.

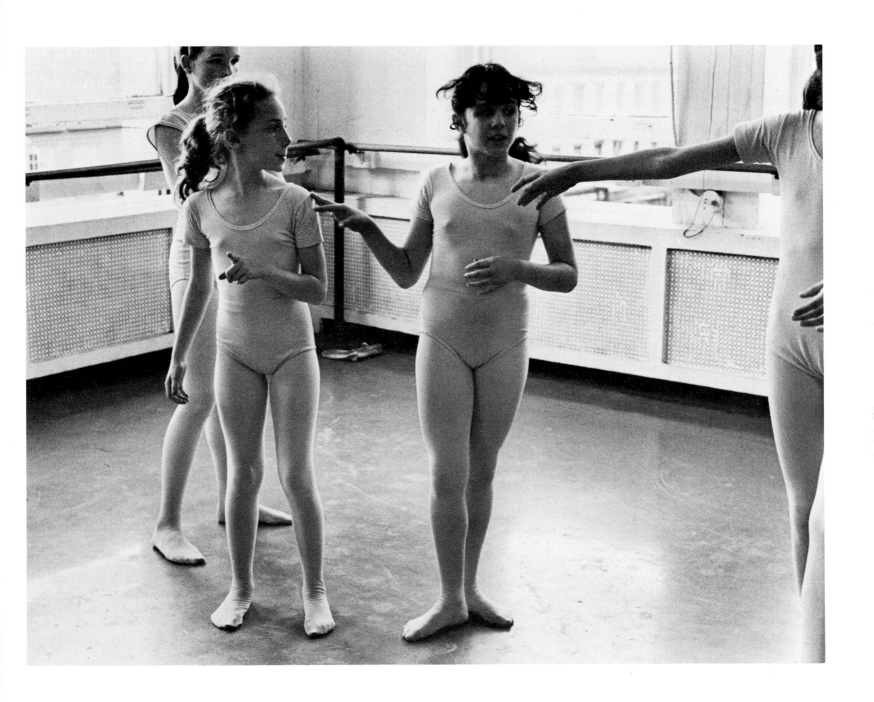

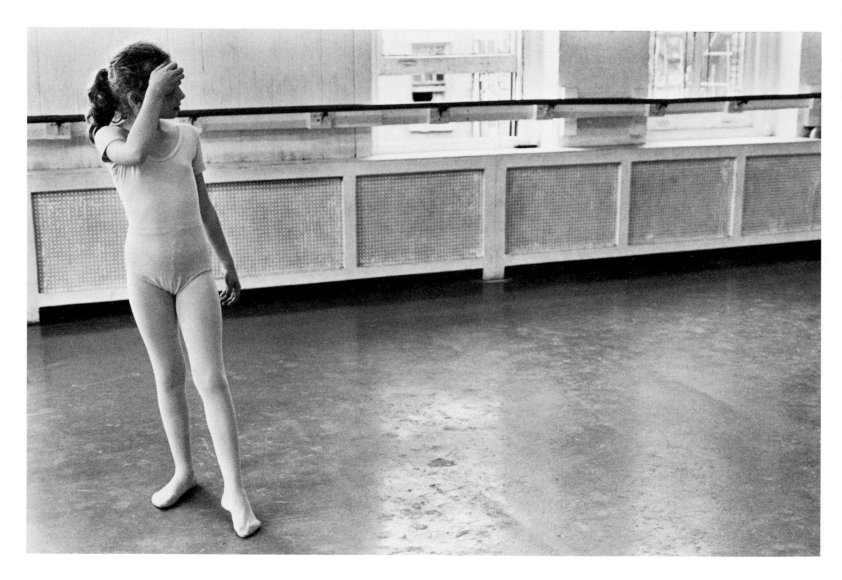

Nancy tries again. This is fun, but it's a challenge, too, spinning by herself so fast down the long room. This time Ms. Baylis applauds Nancy for doing it correctly. Ms. Baylis believes that encouragement brings out the best in every ballet student and that criticism helps a dancer improve. She always

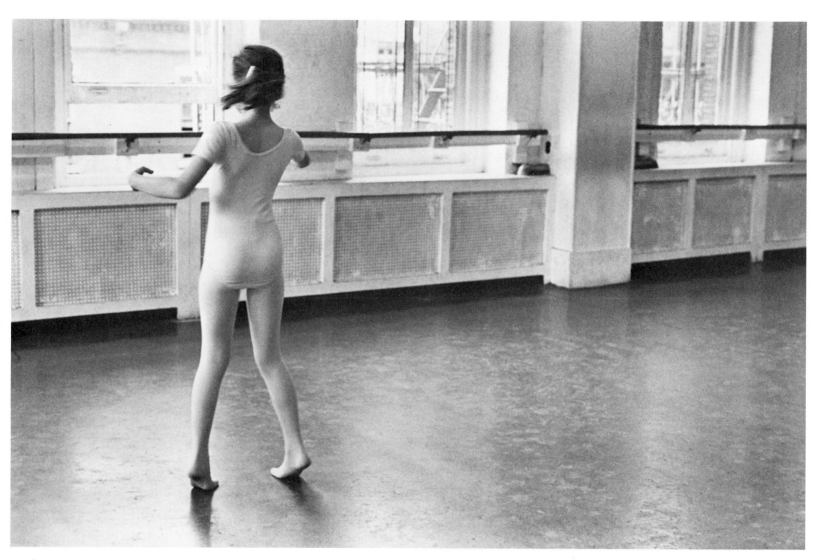

has encouraged all the girls in the class. She says, "To see the girls dance to the music without me is the greatest pleasure I can have, and it makes the girls proud of themselves, too." And this pride makes them work harder.

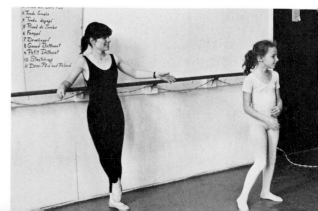

Making sure that all the students' backs are straight, their stomachs in, and their chins up, Ms. Baylis tells the girls to look at themselves in the mirrors. They should not look down because that puts the body out of line. Lauren goes among the students, poking a stomach here and moving a foot there. There is quite a lot of giggling among the girls as they study themselves in the mirrors.

Nancy is having trouble again with the position of her arms. Ms. Baylis comes and shows her in the mirror just how to hold them.

It is all right for the students to make mistakes, because that is the only way they can learn the difference between correct and incorrect positions. But the students are expected to remember their mistakes. Including Nancy, too!

They go through the motions of the *tendu*. Every girl stands in the fifth position, with the right foot out front. The foot is then moved outwards until it becomes firm and well arched, without lifting the toe from the floor. The leg is then moved in an arc outwards as the toe touches the ground. The body weight is always on the opposite leg, and lets the other leg swing freely. It should return to the fifth position without any trouble. This movement is repeated two more times; the second time the right foot goes out sideways, and the third time, the left foot moves out behind, away from the body.

The entire line of students repeats the exercise until Ms. Baylis tells them to stop. She explains that the *tendu* is a good movement for feeling all the joints and parts of the foot.

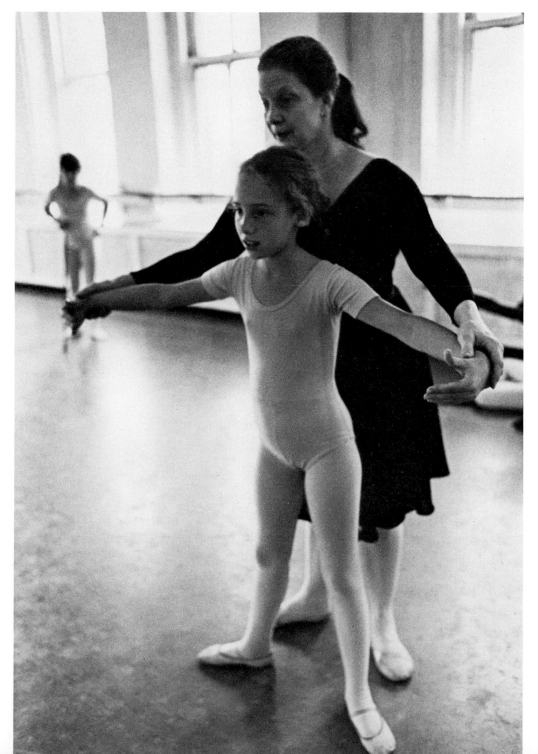

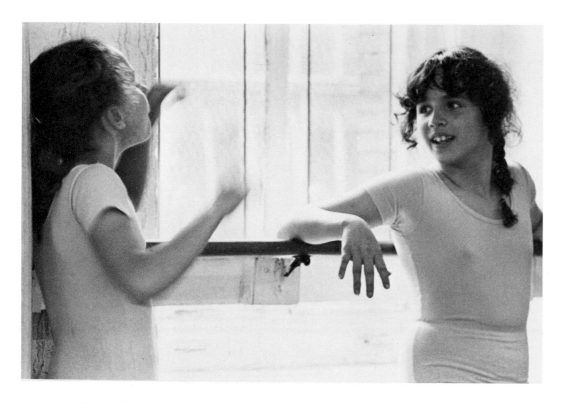

    In ballet class, Nancy has another friend, Debra, with whom she shares secrets. Sometimes they play tricks on their teacher. Nancy tells Debra that she is going to imitate Ms. Baylis behind her back while she is demonstrating a step. Ms. Baylis is unsure if Nancy is behind her, and she has to look behind her back and catch Nancy laughing. Ms. Baylis laughs too.

    But most of the time, the class must be well disciplined so that the students can learn. There is so much to learn. Some of the movements are not easy to do.

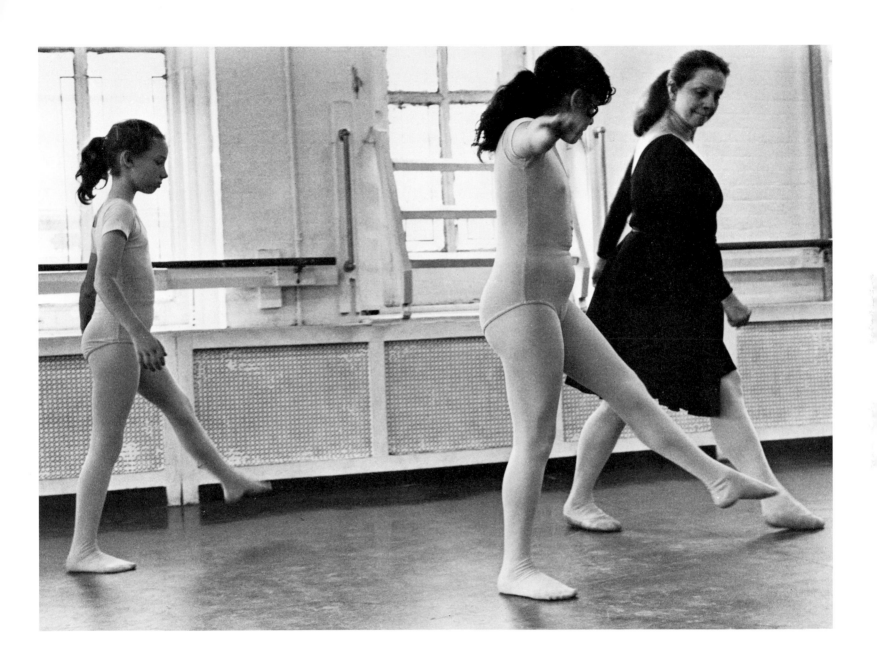

Ms. D'Addario, director of the Joffrey Ballet School, comes into the studio. She says that a TV videotape crew will be coming in a few minutes to videotape the class for a local network news show. The class gets excited. They've been on television before, but they still think it's fun.

Being videotaped does not distract the girls from their weekly practice. They are aware that they must keep working to become successful dancers.

After Ms. D'Addario leaves, Ms. Baylis organizes the girls beside the *barre*. They go through the practice movements of the *demi-plié*.

In French, *demi* means "half" and *plié* means "bend," so a *demi-plié* means that the legs do a half bend. *Pliés* are very important in ballet because they are used in many other movements. In the *demi-plié* the dancer stands in the first position and bends her knees slowly, with her knees turned out and her feet flat on the floor. Then she returns to the standing position. The movement must be done very smoothly. There should be no jerky motions.

The class does the *demi-plié* in the second through fifth positions, their knees bending in the middle of each position.

Then they go through the *grand-plié,* or full bend, exercises. These are the same as the *demi-plié*, except that the dancer bends her knees and moves her body downward, with the knees well out. All five positions are done with the *grand-plié*. The class has many more exercises to do.

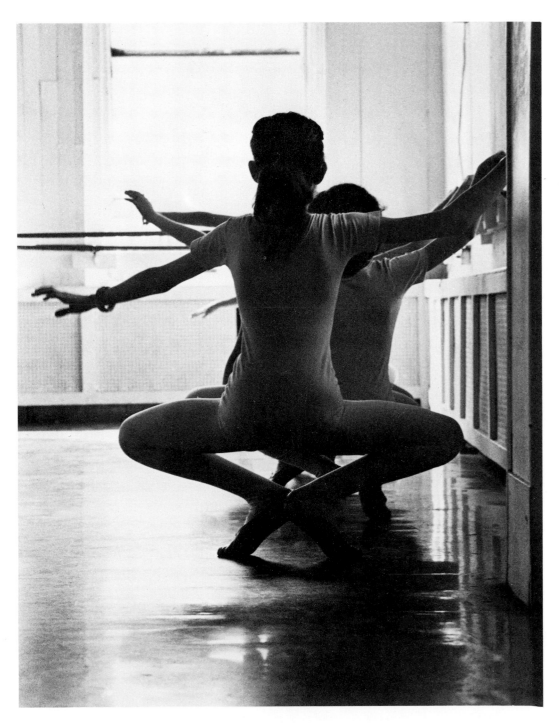

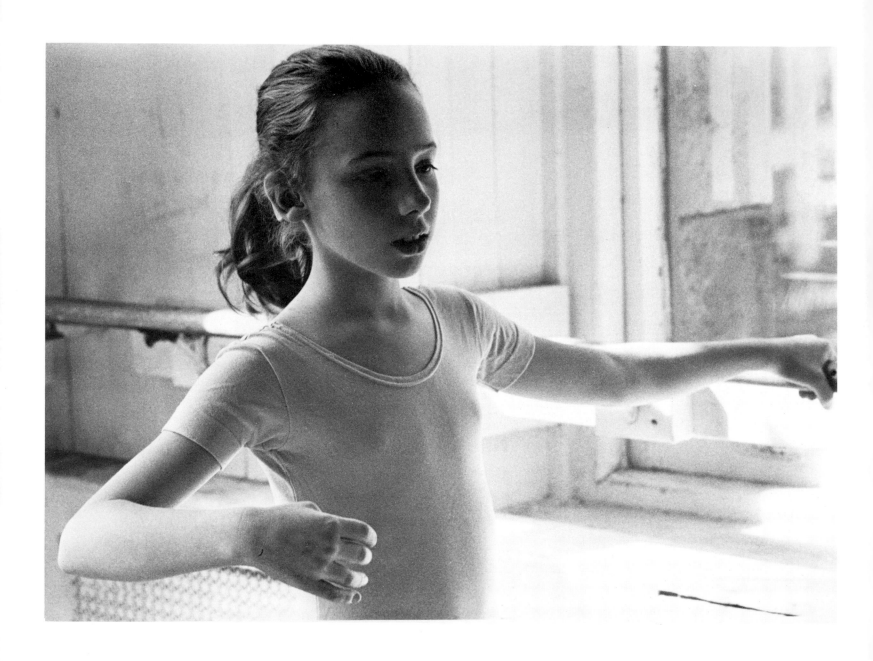

It is very hard work to change to different exercises as we practice, but Ms. Baylis told us it was good because later on, we would have to do the same thing if we were really dancers. We would have to remember what the next dance step would be.

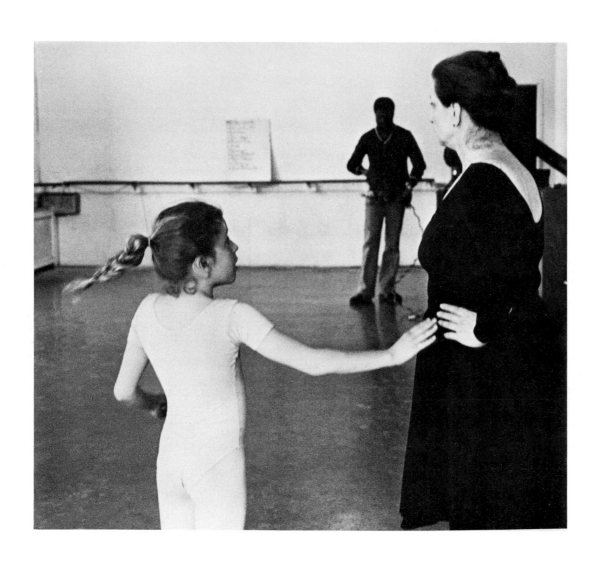

Nancy complains of being tired. Ms. Baylis tells her that many dancers feel tired after a workout. It may mean that she needs some extra sleep. Ballet uses up a lot of energy. Many dancers sleep longer and eat better while rehearsing for a new show, so that they can come to every rehearsal in perfect health. They need a lot of stamina to keep up with rehearsals.

A ballet dancer needs a good clear, alert mind. This is especially true for Nancy and her classmates, because they must rely on their eyes more. When everyone feels rested and alert, the classes run more smoothly.

The TV videotape crew finally arrives. The crew members come bustling in, carrying lights and cameras. Marianne explains to the class how the TV crew will work. The students take a short break, waiting for the crew to set up the bright lights for filming. The light in the studio is not strong enough for videotaping.

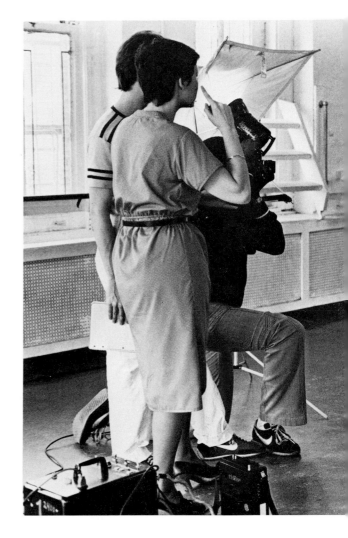

51

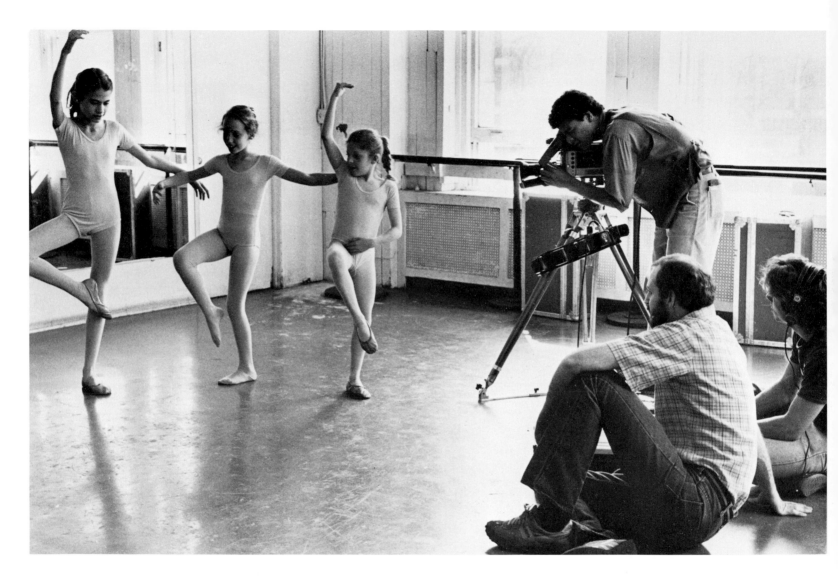

As soon as the lights are set up, the class continues with the exercises. At this point, the class is beginning to look like a group of little ballerinas practicing: pretty, strong, moving on quick feet; a feeling of placement; a nice balance of body.

As the girls go through the other movements, the TV people move around the studio, filming different scenes. One girl stops and tells Ms. Baylis that she cannot do the *arabesque*.

"Whatever makes you say that?" asks Ms. Baylis.

"Because deaf people don't have a sense of balance," the girl answers.

Some deaf people have very poor balance, because of a lack of fluid in the ear canal. This fluid must carry vibrations of sound from the outer ear to the inner ear. When the fluid is missing, there is no sensation of vibration, or the push and pull of sound that helps give a person a sense of balance.

"Can you try again?" Ms. Baylis asks. "Even hearing children have trouble with the *arabesque*. You can learn how to balance. Just look down your nose at your finger and raise your leg!"

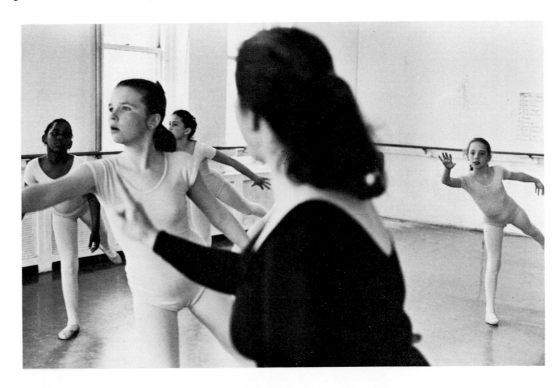

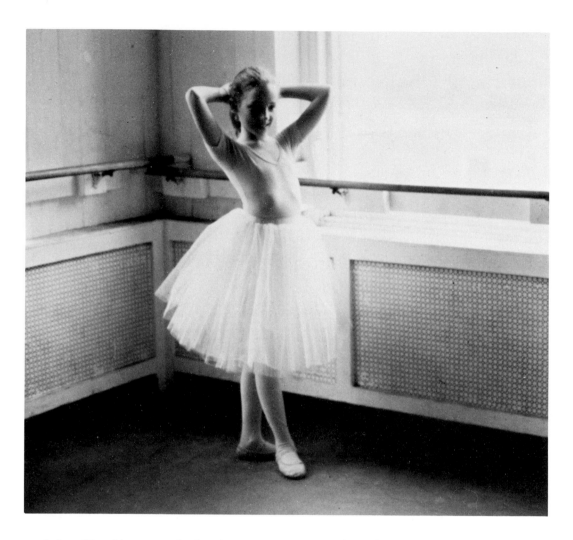

Ms. Baylis says it is time to put on the skirts. "We shall go through all the steps with your skirts on. We must get ready for parents' day." The girls rush to put on the skirts and practice some more before class ends. Wearing their skirts, they feel like real dancers.

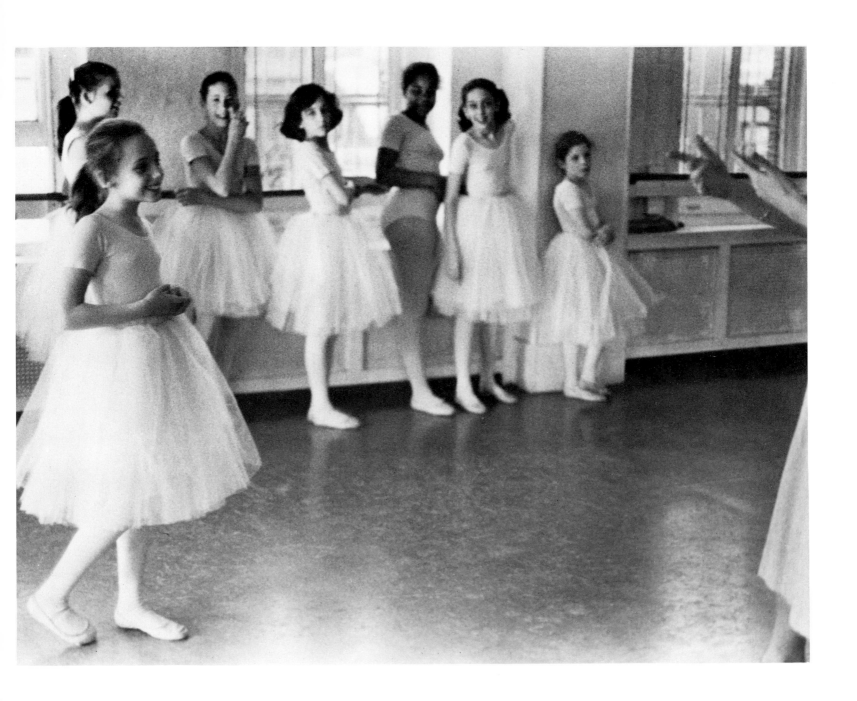

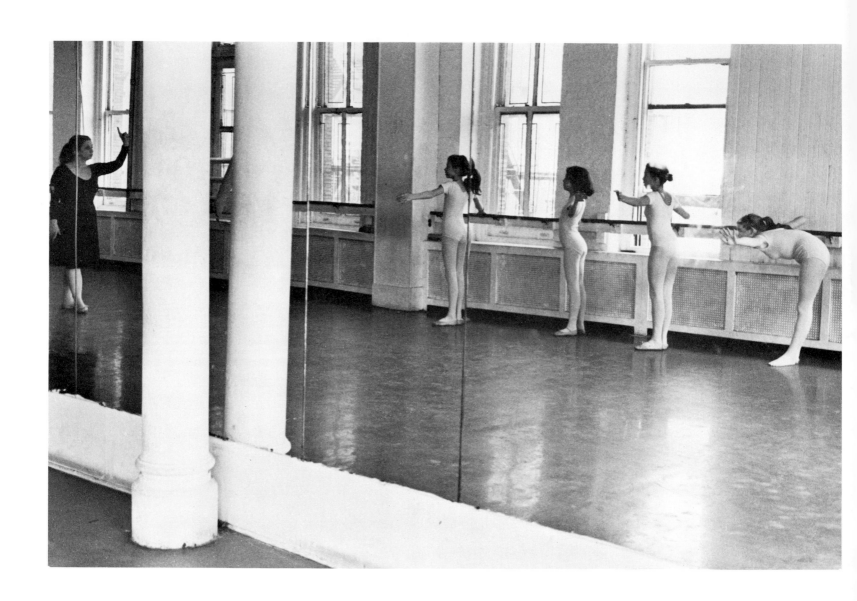

The class ends with stretches, and then each student says thank you to Ms. Baylis for her instruction, and goes out to the dressing room to change. The TV crew asks Nancy to stay behind to be interviewed.

The interviewer asks her if she likes ballet.

"It's fun, and I love it."

"What about the different movements? Can you remember all of them?"

"At first, it was hard. But now I know the right names. And I like them all. They help me to be more graceful. Now I know a little bit more how my body works."

"How do you understand the music? Isn't that difficult?"

"No. My hearing aids help, and I concentrate a lot." Nancy laughs. "And the music that makes me dance is the music I feel!"

"Wonderful! Tell us, Nancy, what is your dream for the future?"

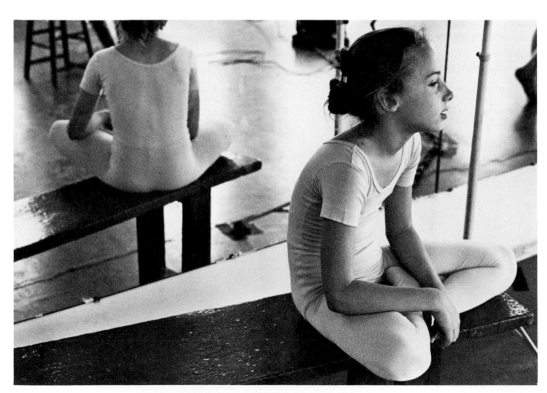

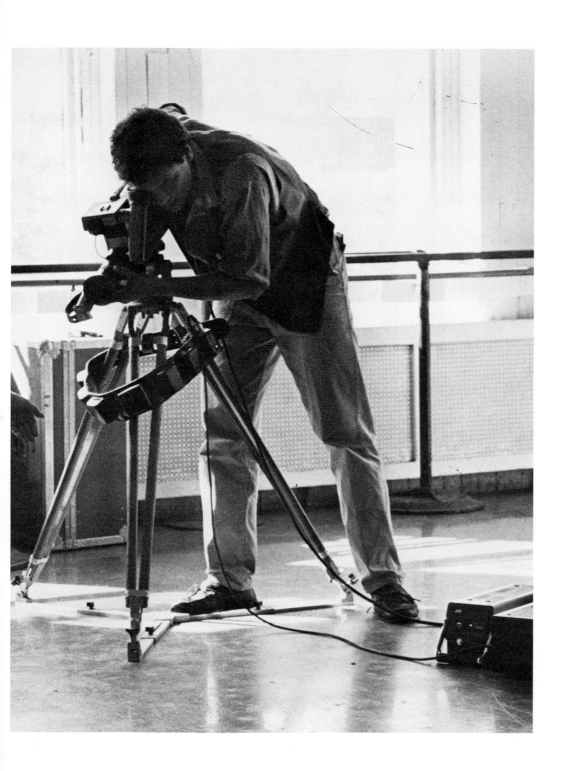

Nancy thinks a minute, and then, remembering, she says, "To dance again at Lincoln Center. I want to be on that stage again. It was so exciting! I want to be a dancer."

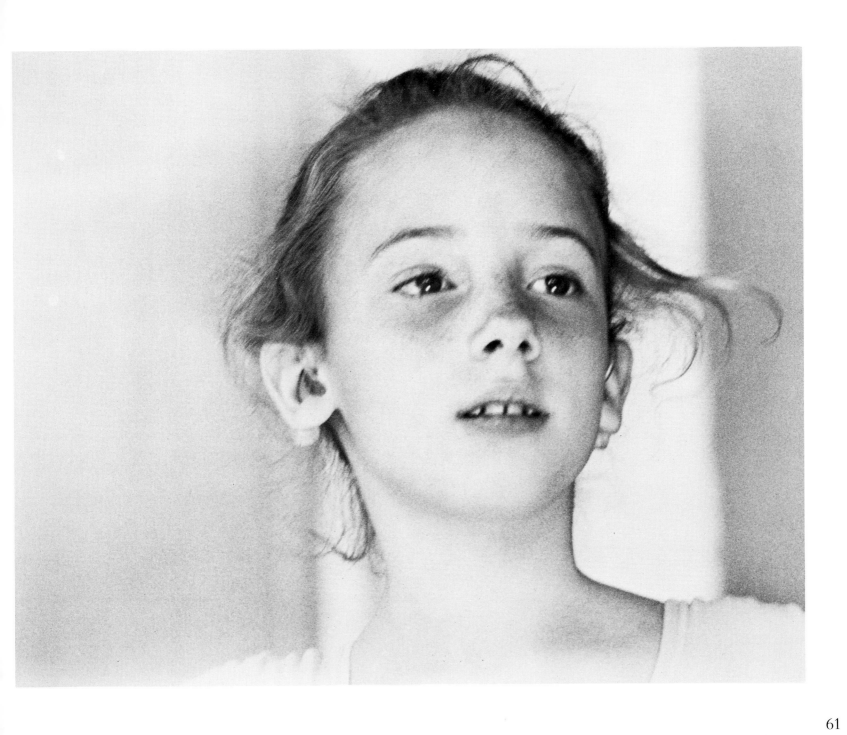

The bright lights are turned off. The cameras are packed away. Nancy goes off to change her clothes in the dressing room. One more whole week until next Friday. And many more weeks of practice—to become a good dancer.

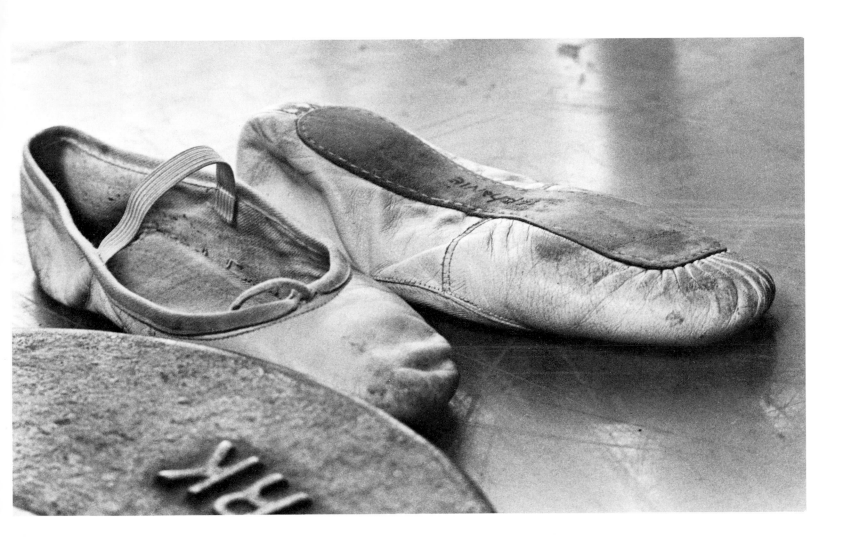

A Word from the Author

I have worked in the show business world as an actor, dancer, director, and playwright, and I am now finishing a degree at New York University.

I first met all the girls of the special class at the Joffrey Ballet School when they and I appeared on the same dance program at Lincoln Center. Ever since then, my interest in the class has grown until I wanted to write a book about it. I decided to write it from the viewpoint of one student, my sister Nancy.

I visited the class on many Friday afternoons, watched them and took notes. On every visit I was amazed at the amount of energy and happiness that the class showed.

I want very much to thank Jane Steltenpohl; Edith D'Addario, director of the Joffrey Ballet School; Meredith Baylis, teacher and friend of the girls in the class; Marianne Gluszak, who makes communication much easier; and Judith Evans, for her work in making the class a reality. I want to express my appreciation for the involvement and enthusiasm of all who made this book possible. And most of all, my thanks to Nancy and her classmates.